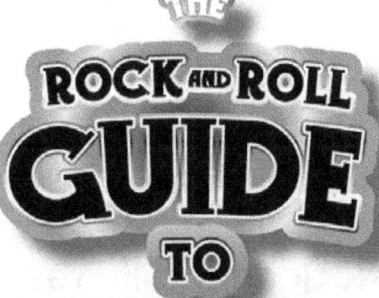

THE ROCK AND ROLL GUIDE TO PATIENT LOYALTY

Joe Heuer

The Rock and Roll Guide to Patient Loyalty

Joe Heuer

Published and distributed in the United States by:

Rock and Roll Press
2435 West Greenwood Road
Glendale, Wisconsin 53209
(414) 247-0936
RockandRollGuru.com

ISBN: 9781439210048

Cover and layout by Douglas Golner

Preface

If you work in health care, this book is for you, no matter what job title is on your identification badge. Creating patient loyalty is the responsibility of every single person in your organization.

The principles that follow are universal. Bring them to life and you will create the environment that leads to patient loyalty.

What do Rock and Roll and Customer Service have in common?

They're both an
ATTITUDE!

Patient Loyalty
from A to D

I was going to do the A to Z guide to patient loyalty, but I decided against it because I couldn't think of anything good for X, Y or Z.

So here is the A to D version. All you need to do is go

Above and

Beyond the

Call of

Duty

Introduction

One Monday morning when my beautiful little girls were three years old, they asked me where I was going and for one of the few times in my life I was speechless. I wasn't about to tell a pair of three-year-olds that I would be out delivering customer service training. They were already at the age where they started looking at me like I was nuts, and I didn't really want to add fuel to that particular fire.

As I sat thinking about how to respond, I realized that if I couldn't explain it to them in a way they would understand, maybe I didn't have a very good grasp of it myself. Suddenly, I had a BFO (Blinding Flash of the Obvious). I've got several 300-page books on customer service sitting on my bookshelves, and I've even read the first chapter of most of them...but it doesn't take 300 pages to explain customer service. It's really quite simple.

In fact, I realized that all we really needed to know about customer service we learned in kindergarten.

Here's the BFO part. Customer service is two simple core principles:

1. Be nice

2. Be helpful

DUH!

That's it. When you break customer service down to its essence, that's all there is. While most kindergartners have mastered these two concepts, the vast majority of organizations run by adults ignore these simple rules.

If you are seeking a more complicated explanation of customer service or patient loyalty, this probably is not the right book for you. There is plenty of boringinformation out there that would better suit your needs. However, if you are genuinely interested in the simple truths of creating patient loyalty (along with a healthy dose of irreverence and sarcasm), keep reading. This book might just become your own profitable little road map to patient loyalty.

Lip-synching:

the rock & roll equivalent of the fake customer service smile.

Patients Are Customers!

There is sometimes a level of discomfort in health care over the term customer. Although our focus is on patient loyalty, you will also see the term customer used for the following reasons.

Customers are, by definition, people who want or need a service that you offer and are willing to pay for it. Therefore, patients are customers. Customer is also a commonly accepted term that refers to more than just your patients. Employees are considered internal customers and they are the foundation of any organization.

Additionally, I'm going to encourage you to take a brief mental vacation from work in order to think about what you like and what you don't like in terms of the customer service you receive in your daily interactions. This should provide you with some clues regarding what your patients like and dislike. Finally, your patients refer to the service you provide as customer service, and their perspective is the only one that determines their loyalty. So deal with it.

Satisfaction:

a customer service term meaning excessively mediocre and something the Rolling Stones could never seem to get.

**Provide the Rockin'
service that makes your
patients say
"WOW!"
or its first cousin,
"KEWL!"**

In the Beginning

Let's start by assessing the level of customer service you most commonly receive in your daily interactions. Begin paying attention to the places you frequent on a regular basis. How do they treat you? Are people nice? Are they helpful?

If you are like most people, you're starting to get a little agitated just thinking about it. I know what you are thinking and you are right…it is pathetic out there. In other words, customer service at most places stinks. Yes, you read correctly…customer service at most businesses is atrocious. Obviously, I've decided not to sugarcoat it.

Whereas this scenario is a real drag for us as customers, the flip side is that you can learn from these experiences and they can help you to develop your own brand of ROCKIN' service that will lead to patient loyalty.

None of this is complicated. It is simple, although not always easy. And it requires you to take action. I think you will agree that is a small price to pay for patient loyalty.

Now think about those places where you are truly loyal. What have those companies done to make you loyal? How do they treat you? More importantly, how do they make you *feel*? If you can't think of a specific company, simply imagine what it would be like to be loyal and then answer the questions.

Don't feel bad if you can't think of anyplace. It's common in my seminars for less than ten percent of the attendees to be able to identify even one company to whom they are loyal. That's just more validation of my premise that service levels are at an all-time low.

The good news is this makes it easier for you to stand out from the crowd and create patient loyalty.

If what you are doing is not creating patient loyalty, it's time for some ch-ch-ch-ch (you know where I'm going with this) **CHANGES!** *Obviously, I was listening to David Bowie when I wrote this.*

The New Competition

Stop worrying about what other health care providers are doing because they are no longer your competition. You read that right. They are no longer your competition if your goal is to create the culture of service excellence that invites patient loyalty.

We know that the overall perception of customer service in health care is not stellar, to put it mildly. If your attention is on other health care providers then you are setting the bar way too low. Start thinking of your competitors as those organizations that are the best in the world at providing top-notch service. This will help you create the mindset that will move you in the direction of becoming a world-class service provider.

The best of the best includes companies such as Disney, Ritz Carlton and Nordstrom. It doesn't matter that they are not in your industry. What matters is that these organizations have created models for service excellence that are unparalleled. The principles of service excellence are universal, which means they transcend industry.

How much patient loyalty would you create if your service culture paralleled Disney's?

If you were put on trial for delivering the Rockin' service that inspires patient loyalty, would a jury have enough evidence to convict you?

What is Loyalty?

What is loyalty? I regularly ask audiences to tell me, in one word, what loyalty is. The responses I hear most often are commitment, responsiveness, great service (okay, so some people don't quite get the concept of one word), dedication and excellence. Those are all certainly components of patient loyalty, but none of them answer the question. In one word, loyalty is a **feeling** or an **emotion**. Make a special note of this because we will be coming back to it repeatedly.

Putting the two together, patient loyalty is a feeling people have about you that inspires them to keep coming back. It is a feeling that also inspires them to encourage their friends, family and colleagues to use your services. Loyal patients do not necessarily do this because of the quality of your service, but because of how they **feel** when they think about their experiences with you.

If you want loyal patients, you gotta blow 'em away with ROCKIN' service!

What do Loyal Patients Do?

Loyal patients would rather fight than switch. (Yes, you really are old if you remember where that phrase came from.) Not only do loyal patients keep coming back, they also become your most effective sales force. Loyal patients tell the world how great you are. Considering that it costs approximately six times more to acquire a new patient than it does to keep an existing one, that is worth more than any advertising or marketing campaign you can undertake.

Loyal patients also tend to be more tolerant of delays and other minor problems. And they are more likely to stay with you even when they change insurance plans and have to pay more out of their own pockets.

Create enough loyal patients and they will be the only sales force you will ever need. Eventually, you will be able to eliminate your entire marketing department. How much money will that save you?

Note to marketing people: that was a joke.

Satisfied Patients

Before we go any further, I need to address a group of people that you have heard so much about. They are the satisfied patients.

Satisfied patients are not the same as loyal patients. Satisfied is a customer service term meaning excessively mediocre.

People who consider themselves merely satisfied report that the will say adios in an instant if they think they will have a better experience elsewhere. Loyal patients will keep coming back even if it is a little less convenient and a little more expensive.

Do you want satisfied or loyal patients?

The Psychology of Patient Loyalty

(the abbreviated version)

Human beings are, first and foremost, creatures of emotion. We make the majority of our decisions based on feelings or emotions. We then attempt to justify those decisions logically. When we make decisions regarding our health care providers, those decisions are almost always based on our feelings.

Obviously, making people feel a certain way is at the heart of the matter. In other words, the heart of the matter really is the heart of the matter.

Are you starting to notice a pattern here?

What Do Patients Want?

Notice that I did not ask what your patients need. I know this may sound a little radical, but please take a moment to focus on what your patients want out of their encounter with you. Your patients want to feel better as a result of having come to you. They want to feel better emotionally as well as physically.

Think about it this way. Most people are not in a particularly good mood when they come to a hospital, clinic or doctor's office. They don't come in skipping and whistling a tune about how delighted they are to be there for a test, procedure or even the run-of-the-mill yearly poking and prodding. Anything you can do to make their visit a positive, or at least less uncomfortable, experience will be greatly appreciated. This is the responsibility of each and every person the patient encounters, from the receptionist to the doctor and everyone in-between.

Remember that positive experiences lead to positive relationships, and positive relationships are the foundation of patient loyalty.

Your patients want a positive experience. Give them one and you'll be on your way to earning their loyalty!

What Else Do Patients Want?

Your patients want you to care. Think of the word care as an acronym for:

Communicate

Attitude

Reliability & **R**espect

Empathy

Communicate simply means to tell people what they need to know in a clear and compassionate manner.

Attitudes are reflected through your interactions with your patients and are an indication of your feelings toward them.

Reliability is doing what you say you are going to do when you say you are going to do it.

Respect is showing proper courtesy. This used to be called common courtesy. Unfortunately, it's not so common anymore.

Empathy is attending to people with your heart.

The Mantra

Patient loyalty begins with me.

Moments of Truth

Every interaction with a patient, whether it is in person, on the telephone, through written correspondence or advertising, is a moment of truth. It is during these moments of truth that loyalty is earned.

Each moment of truth gets stored in the patient's memory bank. Basically, they are making mental notes on the interaction and giving you a check mark in either the positive or negative column. To create patient loyalty, you need to amass a plethora of check marks in the positive column while avoiding the negative column.

The Two Dimensions of Service

There are two dimensions of service: technical and personal. The technical dimension typically relates to quality. A wonderful thing about health care is that you already have this part of the equation mastered, since technical excellence is the price of admission into the marketplace.

Unfortunately, quality is generally not enough to create loyalty. If quality alone determined customer loyalty, how could you possibly explain Domino's Pizza?!?!?

It's really quite simple. Domino's makes people feel good about dealing with them. Even though they have not advertised their "thirty minutes or it's free" guarantee for a number of years, most people still associate Domino's with rapid delivery. They have created the feeling that you can depend on them when you are in a time crunch. In other words, they have mastered the personal dimension of service by creating a positive connection with their customers. And that alone has earned them tremendous customer loyalty.

Your organization has half of the equation mastered through your technical excellence. However, you must cultivate the personal dimension of service if you hope to make the quantum leap from patient satisfaction to patient loyalty.

Keep it Simple

We've already determined that customer service is a simple concept. Be vigilant in keeping it that way, because the process fanatics in your organization will do their best to complicate it as much as humanly possible.

If you're not sure who the process fanatics are, they are the people who always need to do seven more case studies, pilot programs and reengineering on matters as basic as how you answer the telephone. They are usually so wrapped up in systems that they are completely oblivious to the immense impact of the human interaction. Watch out for the process parade at all costs.

Here is a wonderful quote endorsing the simplicity of service:

"Everybody can be great...because anybody can serve. You don't have to have a college degree to serve. You don't have to make the subject and verb agree to serve…you only need a heart full of grace, a soul generated by love."

Martin Luther King, Jr. said that. It doesn't matter that he wasn't talking specifically about customer service. What matters is the essence of this simple message: Anybody can serve.

How much simpler can it get? Earn your patients' loyalty through ROCKIN' service. Be proactive. Do a little something extra, and make their experiences dealing with you memorable. Serve your patients better than anyone else can—it's the one thing in the loyalty equation that is totally under your control.

Think Like a Patient

In the movie Caddyshack, Bill Murray's character was trying, without much success, to catch a gopher that was tearing up the golf course where he worked. In a Blinding Flash of the Obvious he realized that to catch the gopher, he had to think like a gopher.

While I'm not suggesting you think of your patients as gophers (unless you are a veterinarian), there was a method to his madness that is relevant to you. If your goal is to create loyal patients, then start to think like a patient. In other words, put yourself in their shoes.

For example, how do you feel when you are forced to navigate a complicated voice mail system, which is the device of choice for organizations that want to annoy their customers without making the effort to do so live and in person. If you find it annoying, take that as a cue as to what your patients think about it!

Learn to think about the service you provide from the patient's perspective and you'll be well on your way to creating the positive relationships that lead to patient loyalty.

The Great Barrier

"But that's the way we've always done it..." If I had a dollar for every time I've heard that, I'd be off on a yacht in the South Pacific.

TTWWADI (that's the way we've always done it) is truly the great barrier to patient loyalty...with one caveat. If the way you have always done it has created the level of patient loyalty that you desire, hooray! Keep doing what you are doing. However, I doubt that that is the case, because if it were you probably would not be reading this book.

Here's a real complicated concept. If doing things the way you have always done them is not creating patient loyalty, change the way you are doing things. Duh!!!

Treat Every Patient as if They Were Your Grandma

Treat every patient as if they were your own grandma. Would this alter the way you serve? This is one of the questions I always use at the beginning of a training session.

Recently, a manager stopped me during a presentation to ask for clarification regarding whether I was talking about his maternal or paternal grandma. He was obviously unclear on the concept. At that moment I knew it was going to be a very long day.

Typically, when I ask this question most people answer yes. Then I ask them why. The standard response is because they love their grandma.

While it's nice to hear that people love their grandmas, doesn't every human being you encounter deserve the same care, courtesy, compassion, appreciation, understanding, respect and attention you'd give to your loved ones?

If you do not already treat patients this way, give it a shot. If it doesn't work out you can always go back to the way you have always done things.

Patients as Guests

(An addendum to the section on treating every patient as if they were your grandma)

What would happen if you adopted the philosophy of treating your patients like guests? I'd be willing to bet it would increase your chances of earning their loyalty.

You do not have to be in the hospitality industry to treat your patients as guests. By guests I mean people you actually like, not that third-cousin on your mother's second husband's side that always embarrasses everyone and spilled cocktail sauce on your brand new Persian rug.

Treating someone as a guest is simply the art of making people feel welcome and appreciated. Guests are more likely than patients to become friends, and friends tend to be more loyal than patients. Therefore, if you treat your patients like guests, they are more likely to become loyal. I knew that introduction to logic class I took freshman year would pay off someday.

Treating your internal customers like rock stars means more than providing green M&M's and Dom Perignon.

Internal Customers

Internal customers are generally the forgotten customers. Also known as employees, internal customers are absolutely vital to the success of your organization. They are the foundation upon which patient loyalty is built.

You can always get a sense of how an organization will treat you as a patient by observing how the employees treat each other. Brochures and commercials can promise you the moon, but if you notice that people within the organization are treating each other poorly, you can bet that you will be treated poorly, too. Conversely, when employees treat each other well, you can be confident that they will treat you with the care, courtesy and respect you deserve.

This is not rocket science. Treat people well by recognizing and praising their efforts. Consistently let them know that what they are doing is contributing to the overall success of the organization and give them small, unexpected rewards for jobs well done.

In order to earn patient loyalty it is critical that you first earn the loyalty of your co-workers and employees!

I agree with Neil Young that it's very cool to frequent organizations where working people are happy.

Exceeding Expectations

Exceeding expectations is not really the daunting task it appears to be. Consumers have been beaten into submission. Most of the time they are just hoping the experience won't be too much of a hassle. In other words, they have become conditioned to expect pathetic service. Consequently, their expectations are pretty low.

As a customer, that's really a sad state of affairs. On the flip side, it's a terrific opportunity for you as a service provider to distinguish yourself from the crowd. It provides the occasion to use your creativity in order to delight your patients. Do a little something extra or unexpected. My favorite example of someone who exceeds expectations by doing a little something extra is a nurse I know named Bonnie. Whenever she notices that someone is having a particularly bad day, Bonnie provides that person with her anti-depression kit.

It comes in a little bag, complete with a note explaining each of the ingredients. Bonnie's anti-depression kit includes an eraser, so you can make all your mistakes disappear; a penny, so you will never have to say I'm broke; a marble, in case someone says you've lost all your marbles; a rubber band, to stretch yourself beyond your limits; a string, to tie things together when everything falls apart; a hug coupon and a chocolate kiss, to remind you that someone, somewhere cares about you. Do you think Bonnie exceeds people's expectations?

What can you do above and beyond the call of duty in order to exceed your patients' expectations?

Attitude

Every self-help guru in the world spews sermons about attitude and every super-achiever touts the impact of having a positive attitude. Since success tends to leave clues, perhaps this is an area worth exploring.

As a rule of thumb, positive attitudes yield positive results. Lousy attitudes yield lousy results. Again, not rocket science here. Customer service is an attitude, not a department. And there is a huge difference between having a positive attitude and simply having attitude. Most of the places I go I feel like people have attitude.

Much like Disney employees are in character when they greet guests at their theme parks, you are "on stage" whenever you are dealing with patients. They are immediately making judgments about you and the level of service you provide. People who pay attention learn very quickly that a positive attitude goes a long way in dealing with patients.

Better yet, take it to the next level and develop a Rockitude.

Move beyond a positive attitude and develop a ROCKITUDE!

A **ROCKITUDE**

is an attitude that inspires you to act in a manner that brings appreciation, love and joy to every person you encounter!

Passion

Passion is best defined as a persistent preoccupation with an idea others consider unreasonable. Others will tell you it is unreasonable to think you can create a community of wildly loyal patients. They are not necessarily trying to be dream-killers, but they are ignorant. Of course you can do it, but only by exploiting your passion and becoming obsessed with delivering loyalty-inducing service.

Passion will not only help you to serve more effectively, it will bring more energy, enthusiasm and creativity into your life than you ever imagined possible. And passion is contagious. Think about it. Wouldn't you rather be around a person who exudes the fire of passion than one who is just doing a job? Most people view their jobs as places where they work just hard enough to avoid getting fired while getting paid just enough to avoid quitting.

How pleasant is it to do business with these individuals?

Bring the passion of your excitement and enthusiasm to your patients and they will sing your praises to the world. Why? Because passion persuades.

Demonstrate Gratefulness

Thankfulness is one of the pillars of creating patient loyalty. Be genuinely grateful for your patients and you will naturally treat them with a phenomenal level of respect, caring and, dare I say, love.

Be outrageous in demonstrating your love for your patients. It's actually pretty easy to do when you remember that they are the people paying for your kids' education so you don't have to suffer from mal-tuition. They are also paying your mortgage and sponsoring your early retirement. It is not enough to merely feel appreciation and love for your patients. You've got to constantly find little ways to *demonstrate your love and appreciation to them*. Never underestimate the power of a thoughtful thank you.

How do you suppose it would impact your bottom line if your patients knew you loved and appreciated them, felt great about it, and went out and told lots of other people how wonderful you are? You do the math.

Most organizations, even if they really do appreciate their patients, treat it like a well-kept secret. When you realize how hard patients are to come by, it's a no-brainer that you've got to do everything in your power to make them feel appreciated. Small acts of kindness and appreciation can make a huge difference. It takes only a few seconds, yet these acts can help create lifelong patients.

It all comes back to the fact that loyalty is an emotion, and love is the most powerful of emotions. What can you do today, right now, to genuinely demonstrate that love and appreciation for your patients?

Make *EVERY* day a Rockin' patient appreciation day!

Complaints and Service Recovery

One of the fastest and surest ways to assess an organization's commitment to service excellence, or lack thereof, is the manner in which they handle complaints.

People want their complaints handled immediately, if not sooner. Promptness counts. We know that if complaints are resolved at the time they are lodged, and the patient feels good about how the situation was handled, they will likely keep coming back as well as praising you when they tell others how you handled the matter.

Learn to reframe complaints. Think of them as opportunities to improve the level of service you are delivering, since you are learning what the patient thinks you are doing poorly. Additionally, they are giving you a chance to recover and earn their loyalty.

Only a very small percentage of people with complaints will actually tell you, so these patients really are doing you a valuable service. Whether complaining patients become loyal depends on the recovery. If you thrill them with the recovery, they will often forget about the problem.

There are three levels of service recovery: poor, satisfactory and terrific. Poor recovery creates a negative ripple effect, since the patient will probably complain to others about the experience. Satisfactory is the middle ground that elicits minimal response because it reflects excessive mediocrity. Finally, terrific recovery creates the positive ripple effect that leads to patient loyalty.

When the recovery is exceptional, that becomes the focal point of the story that your patient shares with others.

Here's a simple five-step template for service recovery:

1. Thank the patient for alerting you to the problem.

2. Apologize sincerely for the inconvenience.

3. Fix the problem. Acting quickly demonstrates that you have the patient's best interests at heart.

4. Thank the patient for the opportunity to make things right.

5. Follow up. If another department or employee is involved, check to be certain the situation was handled properly.

When handling complaints, also keep in mind what the patient does not want to hear. They don't want to hear excuses. Patients are not interested in hearing about your staffing shortage and they couldn't care less about your computer problems!

Remember, an upset patient can do extensive damage to your reputation, and they rarely hesitate to do so. It's estimated that they tell between eight and twelve people about their negative experiences. Go the extra mile to make things right in their eyes and that is what they will remember.

The Silver Tongue Rule

Communicate with each individual you encounter as if you have to spend the rest of your life with that person in very, very close quarters.

The Loyalty Connection

Your ability to create patient loyalty is directly related to your ability to connect, or establish rapport. Rapport is simply the art of communicating with another person in a manner that allows them to feel connected to you. Concentrate on connecting with individuals as people first, not as patients.

When you create rapport with your patients they will feel good around you. When they feel good around you they will feel good about you. When they feel good about you they are much more likely to become loyal than if they feel indifferent toward you.

The best and quickest way to create rapport is to become a fantastic listener. The key is to take the attention off of you and put it on your patient. Listening makes the other person the star. It also gives you the opportunity to learn as much as possible about your patient's needs.

Listening is an active silence that recognizes the other person's value and makes them feel important. And any time you can make someone feel important, it increases the likelihood that they will become loyal.

As Wilson Mizner said, "A good listener is not only popular everywhere, but after a while he knows something."

Take a breath and actively listen to your patients and you will create the connection that leads to loyalty.

Remember, it is impossible to keep your mind and your mouth open at the same time.

The Greatest Gift

**The greatest gift you can give
to another person is
to be 100% present
in their presence.**

LISTEN

Look at the person

Inquire

Show interest

Tune in

Empathize

Nonverbally respond

The WOW! Factor

When was the last time you were so delighted with the service you received that you said WOW!? Can you ever remember it happening? If it did, I bet you told several people about the experience.

The quickest path to patient loyalty involves uncovering ways to make your patients say "WOW!" or its first cousin, "KEWL!" When you do, they will sing your praises to the world.

Go above and beyond the call of duty and use your creativity to turn the ordinary into the extraordinary.

I once observed a nurse walk into a clinic waiting room and announce, "I'm looking for a nice person named Mary Jones." It put a smile on the face of every single person in that waiting room. Most of us started laughing and a few patients let her know that they were nice people, too. This simple gesture created a WOW! moment while lightening the mood in that waiting room.

Remember, it's the little things that make a big difference. Your patients want to feel like you care about them. Find a way to demonstrate how much you care and you will create the type of memorable moment that makes people say WOW!

How will you use your creativity and personality to make your patients and your internal customers say WOW?

The Power of Humor

You don't need anyone to tell you that working in health care can be an incredibly stressful experience. From a patient's perspective, the experience of walking through your door can be pretty stressful as well. In times of stress, humor is an amazingly effective tool for mentally lightening the load.

I'm not suggesting that you tell jokes or funny stories. Just learn to look at the lighter side of things. It makes life so much more enjoyable for you and for the people you encounter all day long.

Humor is the great equalizer. When you make someone laugh, they feel good. When people feel good around you, they tend to feel good about you. When they feel good about you, they become loyal and tell others about the experience.

Here are two examples of humor that caught my attention.

A sign on the tip jar in a little coffee shop read, "If you fear change, leave it here!" I laughed so hard that I nearly dropped my coffee.

The next one was a sign on the side of a plumbers' truck that read, "A flush always beats a full house." That one put a huge smile on my face.

We all want to deal with people who inspire positive feelings in us, and there is no more pleasurable feeling than laughter. In other words, humor can be a secret weapon that you use to create patient loyalty.

Remember these prophetic words from Jimmy Buffett, "If we couldn't laugh we would all go insane."

Raising the Bar

The mindset for providing exemplary service is one of consistently raising the bar of excellence. Don't panic. This isn't some grandiose plan that requires a comprehensive overhaul of everything you are currently doing.

Raising the bar simply means you focus on elevating your level of service one percent per day. That's it. Anyone can improve one percent. It's such a tiny amount. No one is so good that they can't improve one percent. By improving one percent each day you can multiply your effectiveness in a very short period of time. I used to think that at this rate you could double your effectiveness in one hundred days. That was until I met a banker who labeled me math-deficient while introducing me to the concept of compound interest. He explained that by improving one percent each day it would take only seventy days to improve one hundred percent.

What a concept! You can be twice as good at anything in only ten weeks by improving one measly percent each day. Do you think your patient loyalty would increase exponentially if your level of service was twice as good as it is right now?

What's in it for me?

What's in it for me? (Also known as WIIFM.) It is the most prevalent question most of us ask ourselves on a consistent basis. Why should I be so concerned with providing the top-notch service that leads to patient loyalty?

Frontline employees regularly ask me this question. They often fail to grasp the connection between their personal situation and patient loyalty.

The explanation is elementary, Watson. First, you can't expect to further your own career unless you learn to deliver tremendous service. Second, phenomenal service is always noticed, and you never know who is doing the noticing.

If nothing else, providing fantastic service will lead to the sense of inner fulfillment that can only come from knowing you have helped another person.

That is what's in it for you.

Loyalty is earned by dazzling one patient at a time with Rock Star Treatment!

The Trying Syndrome

Beware of the trying syndrome. Trying is just a noisy way of not doing something. Banish it from your vocabulary right now, or at least catch yourself the next time you hear yourself using it. Simply stop and restate what you are committed to doing, not what you are going to try (and likely fail) to do. As Yoda said in Star Wars, "Do or do not. There is no try." Stop trying and start doing!

Do what you say you are going to do, when you say you are going to do it or you will lose credibility in the eyes of your patient. It's that simple. It's not always easy, but it is simple. Can you afford to lose credibility with your patients?

The 10-Second Customer Service Seminar

Remember that everything you need to know about customer service you learned in kindergarten:

1. Be nice

2. Be helpful

What is Patient Loyalty?

Just checking to see if you have been paying attention. You already know that patient loyalty is a feeling people have about you.

Remember, you can't afford the luxury of having merely satisfied patients because they will leave you in an instant if they think they will have a better experience elsewhere. On the other hand, loyal patients actually pay you for the opportunity to be walking, talking billboards for your services! Is this a great country or what?

ENCORE!

Loyalty will be created only as a result of the actions you take on behalf of your patients. The ultimate success of your business will unfold based on the implementation of these simple principles. Although you can't necessarily control the outcome, you do have total control over your actions.

Your rewards will come not from your knowledge about service excellence, but from what you do with what you know. If you've gotten this far, you already know all you need to know about creating patient loyalty. What you do with it is up to you.

Finally, remember the immortal words of Casey Stengel, "They say it can't be done, but that don't always work."

About the Author

Joe Heuer is known worldwide as the Rock and Roll Guru (RockandRollGuru.com). An entertaining speaker, author and full-time rocker, he shares the nuggets of wisdom he has gleaned from Rock & Roll with professional audiences throughout this third rock from the sun.

He believes that in addition to being a groovy musical genre, Rock & Roll is a way of life that has served as his constant companion and inspiration. Joe has lived numerous dreams, including a stint as the youngest collegiate head basketball coach in the country...who never played the game.

Joe has written several books, some of which have actually been published. His latest book is ***#DreamTweet: Enlightened Inspiration From a Rock and Roll Guru!*** Additionally, ***The NEW Idiot-Proof Guide to Customer Loyalty*** will soon be released in Russian, and he has several other Rock & Roll books in the works.

His wife calls him an idiot savant for his uncanny recall of obscure rock & roll lyrics and trivia.

If you'd like the Rock and Roll Guru, Joe Heuer, to deliver a dynamite presentation for your organization, please contact:

Rock and Roll Guru
(414) 247-0936
RockandRollGuru@gmail.com
RockandRollGuru.com

The Rock and Roll Guide to Patient Loyalty
Special Edition

Create your own special edition of *The Rock and Roll Guide to Patient Loyalty*. Put your organization's name and logo on the front and back covers.

To learn more, please call
the Rock and Roll Guru at
(414) 247-0936

Thank you.
The band has left the building.

www.ingramcontent.com/pod-product-compliance
Lightning Source LLC
Chambersburg PA
CBHW072041190526
45165CB00018B/1324